Controlling Candida Infections

Control the Candida Fungus That Could Be Causing Your Vaginal Infections And Others

RON KNESS

Copyright © 2017 Ron Kness
All rights reserved.

ISBN-13: 978-1545448922
ISBN-10: 1545448922

Contents

Disclaimer

This publication is for informational purposes only and is not intended as medical advice. Medical advice should always be obtained from a qualified medical professional for any health conditions or symptoms associated with them.
Every possible effort has been made in preparing and researching this material. We make no warranties with respect to the accuracy, applicability of its contents or any omissions.

See your healthcare professional before starting any diet, health or exercise program!

Introduction

Anyone who has ever suffered the misery of a Candida infection will know that the best solution to the problem is to prevent it from happening in the first place. Starving Candida, that is, depriving it of the conditions in which it will flourish, is quick and easy once you know how.

In this guide, you will learn what Candida is, what its symptoms are, and which other conditions are linked to it. You will also learn the connection between Candida and digestive issues and discover ways to restore your health naturally, without lots of prescription medications.

So let's get started with what Candida is and what causes it.

What Is Candida?

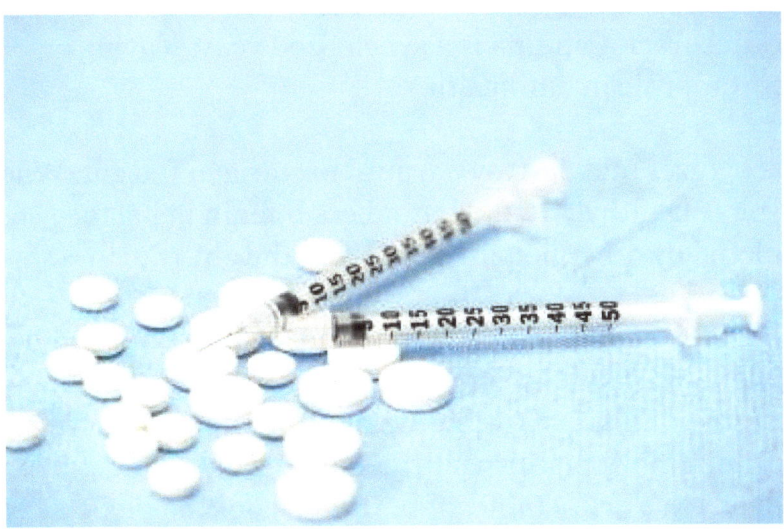

Candida is a form of yeast that lives in the body. There are 20 different species of Candida. However, the most common, and the main one that can result in health issues, is Candida albicans.

An overgrowth of Candida, a condition referred to as candidiasis, can affect these areas of the body, leading to a range of symptoms in the:

- Mouth
- Throat
- Genitourinary tract
- Skin
- Nails
- Intestines
- Blood

Candida may sound horrible and something you want to get rid of completely, but in fact, it is actually a normal part of the gut flora, that is, micro-organisms that live in our digestive tract. Candida is a specialized yeast playing an important role in our health.

It recognizes and destroy harmful bacteria in the gut. When a person is healthy, Candida numbers remain in balance, regulated by other helpful bacteria in the gut.

However, if something causes the gut flora to become imbalanced, Candida can proliferate and change from a *yeast to a fungus*. In the mouth and throat, it is known as thrush. In the genitourinary tract, especially women, it is referred to as a yeast infection. If it invades the blood stream, it is known as invasive Candida. On a baby's bottom, it is known as diaper rash.

Candida As A Fungus
In its fungal form, Candida starts to invade the invasive mucus membranes and intestinal walls in the body. It produces rhizoids, which have a very long root-like structure, which can burrow deep and leave microscopic holes.

These openings allow toxins, undigested food particles and bacteria and yeast to enter the bloodstream. A 'leaky gut' has been cited as the cause of many autoimmune disorders, that is, conditions in which the body starts to attack itself. Therefore, it is important to keep Candida levels normal and not allow for overgrowth.

Causes Of Candida Overgrowth

There are a number of causes of Candida overgrowth. Determining the cause can help treat the infection effectively. The most common causes include:

Antibiotics

These medicines kill off both harmful and helpful bacteria, so they reduce the number of helpful bacteria in the gut and Candida will no longer be regulated properly and will start to multiply exponentially.

Birth control pills

Any change in hormonal activity can lead to Candida imbalance.

Pregnancy

Pregnancy also brings about significant hormonal changes.

Thyroid disorders

The thyroid produces four different hormones that regulate a range of vital bodily functions, including metabolism.

Immune system issues

A person with a weakened immune system is more likely to suffer from Candida changing to its invasive fungal form.

Other medical conditions

Inflammatory bowel disorders can result in an imbalance of Candida.

Chemicals in food and water

If a person eats a lot of convenience foods with artificial sweeteners such as aspartame (NutraSweet™ Equal™, and other chemicals such as monosodium glutamate (MSG) and mercury, an imbalance can result. Chlorine in tap water has been cited as one cause of Candida overgrowth.

Prescription and over the counter medications

Many prescription and over the counter medications can cause an imbalance. These include:

- Steroids - Immunosuppressant drugs that try to reduce the activity of the immune system, such as methotrexate
- Anti-inflammatory medications such as Advil and Motrin - Antacids, acid blockers or proton pump inhibitors that are used over a long period of time, which will interfere with the entire digestive tract
- De-worming medications
- Lifestyle Issues - A high carbohydrate diet, especially one full of refines carbs such as candy, cake and white sugar
- Yeast-products, such as bread, pizza dough
- Alcohol and fermented foods and drinks, like beer and wine
- Frequent constipation
- Frequent diarrhea, which can cause bacterial imbalance and allow Candida to proliferate
- Mold in the environment

Common treatments for Candida

Treatment depends on where the symptoms are. For oral thrush, you will be given antifungal medication and possibly a special mouthwash and perhaps pills you need to dissolve in your mouth.

For genitourinary Candida, there are a number of over the counter creams and vagina suppositories. Sometimes boric acid is recommended, to be used for up to two weeks.

Some women often experience yeast infections. In this case, they should not just treat themselves with over the counter remedies all the time. They should work with their doctor to determine the source of their infections and try to prevent them.

It is important to treat yeast infections in men and women because they can be passed along through sexual activity, including oral sex.

For diaper rash, commercial creams may be used to clear it up and keep it away.

For invasive Candida, which can be a life-threatening illness, doctors will prescribe antifungal medication, orally and possibly intravenously if the infection is severe.

For intestinal Candida infection, there are a range of dietary and other measures you can take to treat the condition, which we will be discussing in more detail in the rest of this guide.

So now that you know the common causes and treatments of Candida, let's look at the symptoms of Candida, and what illnesses have been connected with Candida.

Symptoms and Conditions Linked to Candida

The symptoms of Candida vary depending on the location of the outbreak.

Mouth and Throat

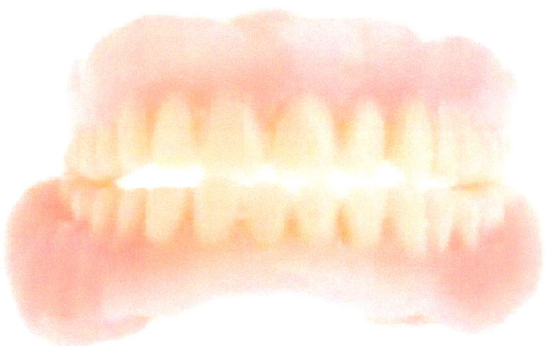

It is important to note that in most cases, a healthy person will not suffer from oral thrush. Those most at risk include those with HIV, diabetes, or cancer. It can also occur in those who wear dentures and don't keep them scrupulously clean. Those who take steroids, post-organ-transplant medications, or broad spectrum antibiotics are most at risk.

The symptoms of oral Candida infection are:
- White spots on the tongue and other oral mucous membranes

- Redness or soreness of the mouth and gums
- Trouble swallowing
- Cracking of the lips and the corners of the mouth, a condition known as angular cheilitis

See your doctor for treatment if any of these symptoms manifest.

Genitourinary tract

A yeast infection can be miserable. Symptoms for men include burning and itching, with the symptoms most acute at the tip of the penis. They might also have a rash all over the penis. It is most common in men who are uncircumcised, so they should pay particular attention to safe sex practices and personal hygiene.

In a woman, the symptoms include:

- Burning
- Extreme itching
- Soreness
- Painful intercourse
- A vaginal discharge that resembles cottage cheese

The symptoms of Candida are similar to those of many other genital infections, so it is important to see your doctor if you have any of these symptoms to determine the exact cause and rule out any sexually transmitted infections.

Diaper rash

Some diaper rashes can be caused by Candida. While most diaper rash is flaming red, diaper rash from Candida looks like dark red patches of skin, particularly in the folds of skin at the tops of the thighs, rather than all over the backside.

You might also notice small yellow pustules that might burst and leave the skin oozing and flaky.

You should always consult a pediatrician before trying to treat diaper rash yourself in order to determine the exact cause and give the right treatment.

Skin and nails
The main symptom is a red, itchy rash, especially in damp, moist areas of the body, such as:
- Underarms
- Groin
- Between the fingers
- Under the breasts
- Skin creases

You might notice small blisters and pustules. The skin can also become dry and cracked, leaving you more prone to Candida invading the bloodstream.

Candida can also cause infections in the nails and cuticles, causing discolored and ridged nails.

Candida resembles a range of other skin conditions, such as eczema and psoriasis, so it is important to get a correct diagnosis from your regular doctor or a dermatologist.

It is important to note that Candida lives even on healthy skin. However, it can become overgrown in certain conditions, such as:
- Warm weather
- Tight clothing

- Synthetic clothing that does not allow air to circulate and the skin to breathe, or for sweat to evaporate
- Poor personal hygiene, such as not bathing or showering regularly
- Not changing your underwear often enough
- Being overweight
- Incomplete drying of damp or wet skin
- Spending too much time in damp clothes such as swimsuits and work out clothing
- Not drying oneself fully after bathing or showering
- Using too many antibacterial soaps

Take steps to keep skin clean and dry. A mild soap and warm water is more than enough to keep skin clean.

Blood

People who develop invasive candidiasis are often already sick from other medical conditions. Therefore, it can be hard to tell if a Candida infection is present. However, the most common symptoms to watch out for are fever and chills despite antibiotic treatment for suspected bacterial infections.

Invasive Candida is particularly dangerous because it can spread to other parts of the body, such as the brain, eyes, heart bones, and/or joints.

Those most at risk are people who have been hospitalized recently, had medical procedures, or are living in a nursing home. Risk factors include:

- The placement of a central venous catheter to give life-saving treatment, such as in an emergency room
- Patients in the intensive care unit (ICU)

- Those with weakened immune systems from HIV, cancer chemotherapy, or organ transplant
- Patients who have diabetes
- People who have kidney failure or are on hemodialysis
- Patients who have had surgery, especially gastrointestinal surgery
- Those who have taken broad-spectrum antibiotics

Conditions linked with Candida overgrowth

There are a number of health conditions linked to Candida overgrowth. According to the Candida Support website, https://www.Candidasupport.org/resources/Candida-related-diseases, these include:

- Irritable Bowel Syndrome (IBS)
- Chronic Sinusitis
- Chronic Fatigue Syndrome (CFS
- Fibromyalgia
- Thrush
- Eczema, or Atopic Dermatitis
- Autism
- Leaky Gut Syndrome
- Crohn's
- Ulcerative Colitis
- Celiac disease

As you can see, most of these conditions are digestive disorders, of a group commonly referred to as Inflammatory Bowel Disease (IBD). Something which is inflamed is red, irritated or swollen. Just think of what your thumb looks like if you hit it with a hammer and you will get an idea of how irritating Candida can be.

A study just published in the journal ***Brain, Behavior, and Immunity*** http://www.sciencedirect.com/science/article/pii/S0889159 116301180 has shown that those with autism who suffer from gastrointestinal disorders have an extreme stress response and produce more cortisol when stress is triggered, which can then lead to a hormonal imbalance and Candida overgrowth. Leaky gut has been linked to CFS, fibromyalgia, and more.

As we have mentioned, Candida exists throughout the body, inside and outside, so it can proliferate on the skin. This can include eczema and other forms of dermatitis, or skin irritation. It has also been connected with acne.

In addition, Candida has also been linked to:
- High Blood Pressure (HBP)
- Attention Deficit Disorder (ADD)
- Attention Deficit Hyperactivity Disorder (ADHD)
- Pre-menstrual syndrome (PMS)
- Prostatitis
- Thyroid issues

Inflammation, or persistent irritation in the body, can cause many of these syndromes.

Candida is also associated with:
- Anxiety
- Depression
- Diabetes
- Earache
- Frequent hunger, even when you have already eaten
- Headache/migraine

- Heartburn
- Insomnia
- Irritability
- Memory issues
- Multiple Sclerosis (MS)
- Muscle pain
- Numbness in the limbs
- Tingling in the arms and legs, hands and feet

The number of behavioral and brain-health issues may be surprising, but new research has shown a very close connect between brain health and gut health, and vice versa, with a two-way connection only just starting to be understood.

A new study published in the journal **Rheumatology** actually showed that brain-related autoimmune disorders could be triggered by altering the gut flora.

This being the case, let's look a bit more closely at how to maintain a healthy gut flora.

Candida and the Digestive System

Candida helps maintain the fine balancing act of the digestive system, killing off bad bacteria and helping good bacteria proliferate. The real danger comes from an imbalance in the gut flora. The imbalance may be caused by stress as well as poor diet and a lack of exercise.

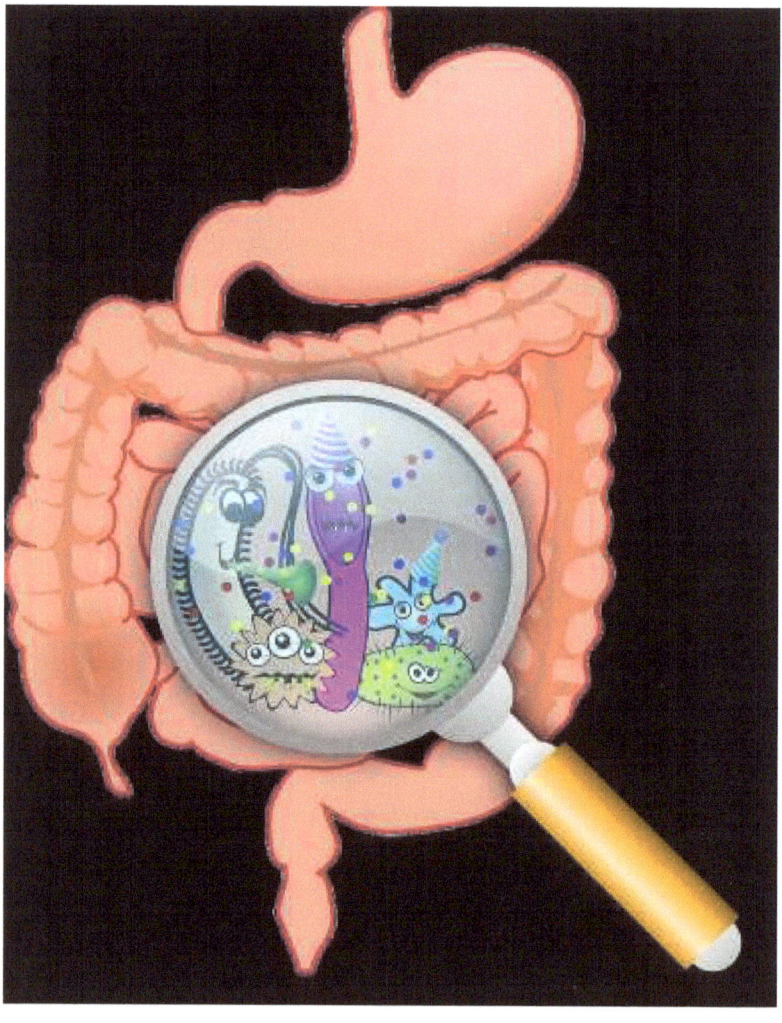

Probiotics

Probiotics are foods which promote healthy gut flora. Yogurt with live, active cultures would be one example. The trouble with many yogurts, however, is they are loaded with sugar. Investing in your own yogurt maker means you can whip it up yourself for pennies compared to commercial brands and eat it with fresh fruit, not sugary substances that needed to be stirred up from the bottom of the yogurt tub.

Probiotics can also be found in the refrigerator section of good health food stores, but they often cost a good deal compared with yogurt and an overall healthy diet.

Prebiotics

Most people know about probiotics, but not many are familiar yet with the fact that probiotics need to eat. Prebiotics are basically the foods sources of the bacteria, to help them thrive. Too many prebiotics, however, can cause proliferation. For example, some carbohydrates are needed for probiotics to eat, but too much can lead to Candida overgrowth.

The average American eats about 300 grams of carbohydrates per day. The Atkins diet allows from 20 to 80, depending on which phase of the diet you are on, so this will give you a good idea of just how many excess carbs people are eating.

Antibiotics

Antibiotics can be helpful in eliminating harmful bacteria, but they kill indiscriminately. In particular, what are termed broad-spectrum antibiotics pose the most risk because they are designed to kill off the largest number of types of bacteria, in a 'scattershot' approach to try to eliminate the one or more bacteria which might be causing symptoms, but leave a person prone to other illnesses as a result.

Over-prescribing of antibiotics, and over-use of broad spectrum antibiotics, is a serious health issue experts are only now beginning to understand the consequences of. Be sure to ask the doctor what kind you are taking and why, and take only as directed.

A course of antibiotics can have a serious impact on gut flora. One study showed that the gut flora, also referred to as the microbiome, had still not been fully restored to balance in some patients two years after they had been taken.

Any course of antibiotics should be followed with a focus on probiotics. Prebiotics should be consumed in moderation.

Probiotics include:
- Miso, as in miso soup
- Tofu/tempeh, which is fermented tofu
- Kefir, fermented goat's milk
- Sauerkraut
- Kimchi (Korean pickled vegetables)
- Apple cider vinegar
- Olives cured in vinegar

Prebiotics include:
- Allium vegetables, such as garlic, onions and leeks
- Dandelion greens
- Asparagus
- Chickory root
- Jicama (pronounced HEE-kah-mah)
- Bananas that have not fully ripened

However, it is important to note that those who adopt a 'Candida diet' are often told to avoid some of these foods, especially fermented ones, and those with vinegar. So what is best?

The truth is there is no one-size fits all Candida diet because people get Candida overgrowth for various reasons and no two diets or sets of environmental circumstance (such as exposure to mold, mildew, chemicals and other allergens and irritants) is going to be the same.

We will outline suggestions for restoring a healthy gut in a moment. But there are three other key elements that contribute to your digestive health which should not be ignored.

Exercise
Exercise is an important part of your overall health. In particular that helps with digestive issues because it helps move things along in the bowel. If you have ever taken a dog for a walk, you will get the idea of how beneficial it can be to take regular exercise in order to eliminate toxins from the body.

Stress management

Lowering stress is always a good thing, but in particular, it has been shown to have significant benefits in terms of digestive health. Not all ulcers are caused by an overabundance of stomach acid due to stress. In fact, about 70% of ulcers are actually caused by the bacteria H pylori.

However, the symptoms of an ulcer can be exacerbated by a lot of stress. If you are not already practicing stress management in your daily life, try to find ways of relaxing and reducing your mind chatter, such as exercise, meditation, visualization, a warm bath and doing things you enjoy.

Good sleep habits

A good night's sleep is essential for your health and weight. Eight hours of high-quality sleep are best in order to restore and renew body and mind after all the wear and tear it has gone through during the day.

Unfortunately, many people suffer from sleep deprivation due to poor sleep habits as a result of too much work, too much TV watching and/or a sedentary lifestyle that doesn't make them sufficiently tired at the end of the day to fall asleep easily. Depression, anxiety, and high stress levels can all contribute to a poor night's sleep.

If you are suffering in any of these areas, exercise such as walking, yoga, swimming and tai chi help with all three issues, bring you back into balance and improving your digestive health at the same time.

Now that you understand what a fine balancing act it can be to maintain a healthy gut, let's look at how to restore it naturally through making smarter choices about the foods we eat.

Return to a Healthy Gut

There are three key steps to restoring healthy gut flora and Candida balance. They are:

- antifungal
- probiotic
- preventive

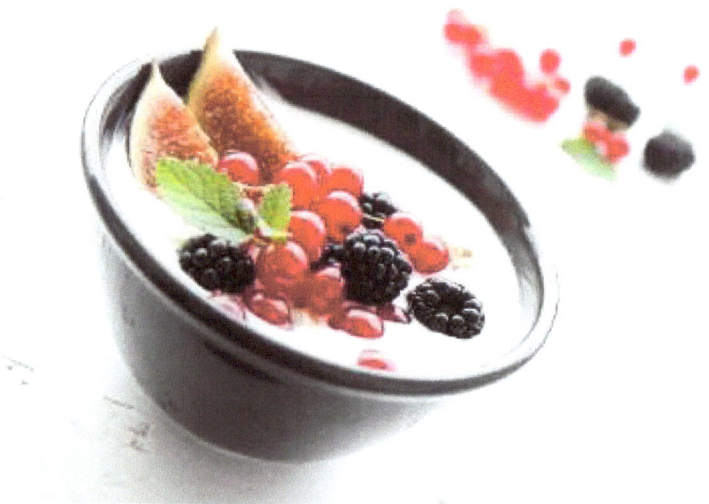

In most cases, your doctor will recommend an antifungal cream or oral medication. You need to use it as instructed to clear up the fungal infection. Once it is cleared up, you can prevent it from gaining a foothold by ensuring your gut is in balance.

Antifungal foods

Those who practice traditional Indian, or Ayurvedic medicine, have recommended various herbs, spices, foods and oils to help cure fungal infections.

Top foods to add to your diet include:
- Ginger-a well-known antifungal, antibacterial and anti-inflammatory root that adds flavor to any dish
- Garlic
- Onions
- Yogurt
- Kefir
- Lassi, an Indian yogurt-based drink
- Kimchi
- Coconut oil

Many of these foods are prebiotic or probiotic as well as antifungal, so they offer a double benefit. Coconut oil is one of the latest food fads. While it is antifungal, it should be used with caution. You should buy only extra virgin coconut oil extracted by pressing in the traditional manner.

You should also only consume it in very small amounts until you can tolerate it well, otherwise it can lead to severe stomach upset. As with all oils, use sparingly, because they are high in fat.

Coconut oil is also very high in medium chain triglycerides, a saturated fat that is supposed to be healthier than long chain triglycerides, but research continues to see exactly how healthy it can be. It certainly adds a lot of flavor to recipes and has soothing anti-inflammatory effects.

Other foods you should add to your diet for their antifungal and 'super food' health benefits include the cruciferous vegetables such as:

- Broccoli
- Cabbage - one study from 2011 linked cabbage to the suppression of Candida overgrowth
- Cauliflower
- Brussels sprouts
- Collard greens
- Kale

Broccoli and kale are considered super foods because they are so packed with nutrition that they are believed to ward off a wide range of diseases.

Pomegranates are also thought to ward off fungus. Be careful with commercial products, however, as they can be loaded with sugar.

Foods which encourage the free passage of toxins through the bowel can also be helpful, and can include figs, prunes, rhubarb and pumpkin seeds. Be careful of the first two, however, because they not only have an extreme laxative effect, they can also contain a great deal of sugar.

Many people attempt a detox, that is, detoxification diet, in an effort to wean them off the bad foods they eat and flush out toxins. Some will also do a colon cleanse.

A detox diet with only clear homemade soups, fresh water and lemon water for 3 days can clear out a lot of issues quickly. Onion soup or cabbage soup will be ideal.

After that, eating antifungals and probiotics regularly should help restore your gut health.

Note: The killing off of large amounts of Candida can result in a Jarisch-Herxheimer Reaction, often called a Herx for short, which means you can feel a lot worse for a couple of days before you start to feel better.

Probiotics

As we mentioned above, it is fortunate that many of the antifungal foods recommended also happen to be prebiotics or probiotics as well. Working out recipes in which all these foods can be incorporated each day can be tricky, but it can also be a food adventure.

For example, Indian food is full of succulent spices. It is also vegetarian and sometimes vegan if you skip the lassi and the fermented Indian cheese known as paneer. They eat a range of pickled and preserved vegetables, and tasty chutneys. Just watch out for the sugar content in sweet chutneys like mango.

Chinese and Korean cooking is mainly based around stir fried vegetables, with ginger as a dominant spice. The great thing about stir fries is you can combine vegetables in lots of different ways, and it takes a very short amount of time to cook.

If you've been living on a lot of packaged convenience foods, this could be one of the reasons for your Candida overgrowth. The trouble with any commercial products is that they are often loaded with sugar, salt and preservatives.

So if you can make your own yogurt and cook dishes such as Indian or Asian dishes, by yourself from scratch, you should soon see a difference in your digestive health.

Supplements

There is a growing number of probiotic and herbal supplements coming on the market, but as with any other kind of supplement, it is a case of buyer beware. Many of these claims have no clinical data to back them up and there is no known dosage. Because these supplements are neither foods nor drugs, they are not regulated by the US Food and Drug Administration (FDA).

Having said that, there are a few herbs and supplements that have shown some promise. These include:

- Cinnamon
- Cloves
- Pau D'arco, taken in the form of tea

Pau D'arco is a South American tree. The name is Portuguese and means 'bow stick' because the wood was used by the indigenous people to make bows for hunting.'

Pau D'arco is said to offer a range of healing properties, including:

- Reducing pain
- Decreasing inflammation
- Antiviral properties
- Antifungal properties
- Detoxifying the body
- Healing stomach ulcers
- Fighting cancer

And of course, treating Candida infections.

However, it should only be taken internally in small doses. It can be applied topically to the skin for the relief of Candida infections there.

Prevention

Once you have added antifungal and probiotic foods to your diet, you should be well on your way to healing your digestive system. Then it becomes a question of what you should eat, and what you should avoid.

An anti-inflammatory diet

An anti-inflammatory diet is one which avoids foods known to cause inflammation in the body, and adds foods know to soothe inflammation.

The most inflammatory foods that should be avoided include:

- Sugar
- Salt
- Fried food
- Cheap vegetable oils
- White flour
- Full-fat dairy such as butter, milk and cheese
- Artificial sweeteners and sugar substitutes
- Artificial coloring, flavoring and preservatives
- Saturated fats, such as from animal products
- Meat from grain-fed animals, such as beef, pork and chicken
- Process meats such as luncheon meat, bologna, hot dogs and bacon-they are full of salt, sugar, nitrites and nitrates

- Gluten, such as in bread, cake and pizza dough
- Trans fats, that is, trans fatty acids, which are (often cheap) oils that have been processed with hydrogen molecules to make them solid and shelf-stable so they won't spoil while they sit in the supermarket for months
- Alcohol such as beer and wine

Foods that have been show to help reduce systemic inflammation in the body include:
- Green leafy vegetables, including Swiss chard and kale
- Bok choy, also known as Chinese cabbage
- Celery and celery seeds'
- Beets
- Broccoli
- Berries
- Pineapple
- Salmon
- Walnuts
- Olive oil
- Ginger
- Coconut oil
- Flax seed
- Chia seeds-also good for bowel regularity
- Turmeric-a bright yellow Indian spice with a mild flavor that adds color and taste to rice dishes

Many people favor what is termed the Mediterranean diet, rich in vegetables and olive oil, with small quantities of high-quality protein such as salmon, beans and legumes. It is an easy way to eat an anti-inflammatory diet if you don't want to spend a lot of time researching what to eat and not to eat.

It is important to note that the traditional Candida diet limits all sweet foods, including fruits like blueberries and pineapple, so it is a good idea to eat them only in moderation and to use as your dessert when you are craving something sweet.

Chia seeds actually make an excellent chocolate pudding as well if you find you can't live without a decadent dessert every so often.

A diet to help with leaky gut

Because fungal Candida burrows into the mucus membranes and intestines, a diet that helps repair a leaky gut might also be helpful.

All of the foods listed in reference to causing inflammation above are on the 'do not eat list' for treating leaky gut. Here is list of the "good" foods you should be eating:

- Olive Oil (Extra virgin if you don't mind the stronger taste)-it is a fat so it should be used sparingly, but it has no cholesterol. Regular olive oil can be used as a substitute for most recipes calling for butter or margarine
- Cherries, sweet, and tart (highly recommended if you have arthritis)
- Walnuts and other tree nuts (if you are not allergic)
- Bell peppers, such as green, red and yellow
- Ginger, fresh root or dried
- Turmeric, fresh root or dried
- Berries such as blueberries, raspberries and strawberries
- Probiotics such as yogurt with live cultures and kefir
- Salmon and Other Fatty Fish with Omega-3 fatty acids

- Non-fish sources of Omega-3s, such as flax seed, tofu, spinach and walnuts
- Green leafy vegetables of any type, such as spinach,
- Crucierous vegetables, such as broccoli and kale
- Bone broth, that is, animal bones like a chicken carcass simmered for 12 to 24 hours with apple cider vinegar until all the nutrition has leached from the bones. It can be drunk as is or used a base for soups and stews.

Now that you know what to eat to restore the health of your gut, let's look at what NOT to eat to ensure a healthy gut and try to prevent Candida outbreaks.

Foods to Avoid During Gut Rejuvenation

There are many foods that can help you improve your gut health, but there are also a few that should be avoided if you want to bring your Candida back into balance so you won't suffer from the infections triggered by an overgrowth.

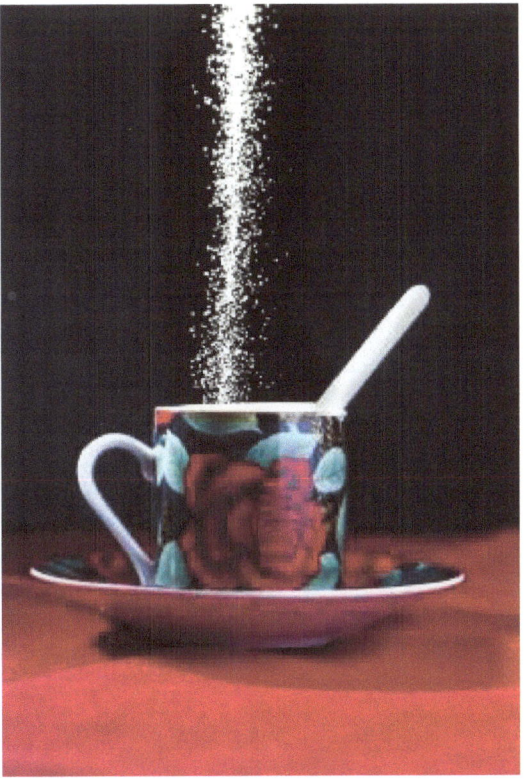

The traditional Candida works on the principle that you should starve the Candida of any chance to proliferate. However, the main problem with this is that the diet is not always sustainable.

Sooner or later, you will either 'cheat', or try to eat like a normal person again, once more adopting a typical American lifestyle in which adults consume about 22 teaspoons of sugar per day. The current recommendation from the American Heart Association is that women should eat no more than 6, and men no more than 9. That being the case, a low carb diet can help.

The list for foods to avoid on a Candida diet are pretty prohibitive for most Americans. The following are NOT allowed:

- Sugar
- Foods raised with yeast, such as bread, pizza dough, rolls
- Fruit juices-they are too sugary
- Dried fruit
- White flour and most wheat products or items that contain gluten
- Full-fat dairy such as butter, milk and cheese
- Artificial sweeteners and sugar substitutes
- Artificial coloring, flavoring and preservatives
- Saturated fats, such as from animal products
- Meat from grain-fed animals, such as beef, pork and chicken
- Processed meats
- Fermented foods like cheese
- Any moldy foods, like bleu cheese
- Fungi such as mushrooms
- Leftovers that have been in the fridge more than 24 hours, since they can start to get moldy on a microscopic level-freeze after cooking if at all possible, or make small quantities

- Unpackaged sprouts and tofu sitting in water in the supermarket-they can be moldy and contaminated with all sorts of things as they sit out in the open uncovered
- Starchy vegetable like potatoes, sweet potatoes and yams
- White pasta, white rice
- Trans fats
- Alcohol such as beer and wine
- Tap water
- Soda of any kind - the regular has too much sugar and the diet has too many chemicals
- Caffeine - it can kill up to 75% of the friendly bacteria in the colon per cup of tea or coffee, or a soft drink containing caffeine, such as Coke or Sprite. It can take about 5 hours for the balance of gut flora to be restored after consuming caffeine.

FAQs About Candida Yeast Infections

The most common question and comment concerning Candida is, *"What is that? I have never heard of that. Wait a minute, isn't that the name of that new pop singer?"* All kidding aside, most people don't know what the word Candida refers to. If you say yeast infection, people immediately think a female-related condition of the vagina.

While Candida does affect many more women than men, it is not gender specific. This fungal infection can affect women, men, the elderly, and children as well as adults. It presents itself in the mouth, the throat, on the skin, on and around the genitals and even in your gastrointestinal tract.

Unfortunately, even though Candida affects as many as 1 in every 3 people, it is vastly misunderstood, even unknown, and often misdiagnosed. Left untreated this yeast infection can lead to bigger problems, including overweight and obesity, diabetes, cancer and other problematic health concerns. Let's take a look at the most frequently asked questions regarding this misunderstood and invasive condition that may just be the underlying cause of many of your health problems.

Q: Why Haven't I Heard about Candida, If It Is So Widespread?

A: Candida Albicans is the scientific name for the yeast overgrowth we refer to simply as Candida. Many people wonder why they have never heard about Candida.

This is because it has only been recognized and well defined clinically for about 30 years.

Since it presents through so many different symptoms, traditionally educated and trained doctors often see Candida symptoms as arriving from some misdiagnosed condition. Candida experts will tell you that most physicians are still battling a learning curve when it comes to recognizing and diagnosing Candida, as well as treating it.

Q: What Exactly is Candida?

A: Candida is a yeast-like, parasitic fungus. It lives naturally in every human being. When your immune system and other physiological processes like your digestive tract are healthy and working properly, Candida is kept in check. A problem occurs when your gut and immune system are compromised.

In this case, Candida grows rapidly, and overgrowth may occur. Candida is a normal part of the flora in your mouth, skin and intestines and a woman's vagina. However, when it runs out of control it can lead to a variety of infections, diseases and health problems.

Q: Who Is Most at Risk for Developing Candida?

A: The following list shows conditions and behaviors that create a higher than average risk for developing Candida:
- Uncontrolled diabetes
- An impaired, weakened immune system
- High levels of sexual activity
- Raised estrogen levels
- Use of antibiotics

- Poor prenatal and infant nutrition
- Vaccinations
- Eating predominantly fast foods and processed foods
- Not enough fiber in the diet
- Not drinking enough water
- Some birth-control medications
- Poor sleep habits
- High stress levels

You can see from the above list that just about anything that compromises your immune system raises your chances of developing a yeast infection somewhere in your body. Women are 7 to 8 times more likely to develop Candida than men. Newborns can contract Candida, if it is present in the mother at the time of birth. Infants and moms can pass Candida back-and-forth via breast-feeding.

Q: Can Men and Children Develop Candida?

A: This was answered earlier, but it needs to be addressed specifically. Yes, men can and do experience yeast infections. These can present themselves in the form of oral thrush, skin irritations, ringworm, jock itch, athlete's foot and display a wide variety of symptoms. Man, woman or child, if you experience poor gut health and/or a weakened immune system, you are at high risk for Candida.

Q: How Do Antibiotics and Other Medicines Cause Candida Infections?

A: Many medications, including antibiotics, attack the bacteria in your body. However, they take no prisoners, and don't know how to recognize good bacteria from bad. So they simply destroy all of the bacteria they encounter, even the good bacteria whose job is to keep Candida under control. This is how some medications raise your risk of developing a yeast infection.

Q: Does Candida Go Away on Its Own, and If so, How Long Before Symptoms Disappear?

A: Over-the-counter medications and natural treatments can return Candida to a natural, healthy level in a week or two in minor cases. If you are on medication or antibiotics, you are constantly killing healthy bacteria, and this can slow down successful treatment. A combination of smart dieting, exercise, hydration and over-the-counter Candida treatments will deliver the fastest results.

Q: What Are the Signs or Symptoms of Candida Overgrowth?

A: The Candida yeast infection can appear as a curd-like discharge that is white or gray in color on and in the genital area. It can also appear as lesions or red, rash-like skin disorders. In the mouth, the tongue or roof of the mouth may develop a white coat. However, when Candida overgrowth is allowed an extended period of time to grow untreated, the symptoms begin to mimic other health concerns.

This could lead to symptoms that mirror diarrhea and constipation, anxiety and depression, urinary tract infractions, heart palpitations, trouble concentrating, irritable bowel syndrome, multiple sclerosis, chronic fatigue and other problems. Menstrual irregularities, loss of sex drive, food allergies and carbohydrate craving, bloating, flatulence and gas, stiff, aching muscles and joints and multiple skin conditions are often symptoms as well.

Children may be diagnosed with ADD or ADHD when a chronic Candida overgrowth is the real cause of the problem. This is why Candida yeast infections are so often misdiagnosed. The treatment is improper so the condition continues to grow, often creating even more health problems.

Q: How Can I Test to See If I Have Candida?

A: Pull up your favorite search engine. Type in "Candida yeast infection online quiz" or some variation of that phrase. This is a quick way to see if you should consult a physician for more extensive and accurate testing. There are spit tests, itch tests and craving tests you can perform at home.

The spit test is simple. Each morning upon rising, spit into a glass of clear water. Is the spit cloudy? Does it form tendrils? Does it suspend itself in the water or quickly sink? If so, you may have a problem. Your doctor can perform urine, blood and stool sample tests as well.

Q: What About the Elderly, Can They Develop Candida?

A: Remember that Candida thrives when the body's natural defense system weakens. The elderly, and for that matter anyone over 50 years of age, has a naturally weaker immune system than when they were younger. Also, since the elderly naturally are more inclined to be taking medications and antibiotics, this additionally raises the risk that they will develop some type of yeast infection.

Q: Can Candida Overgrowth Kill You?

A: Except for very extreme cases Candida is treatable and preventable, and even chronic Candida overgrowth is not deadly. However, candidemia is a dangerous condition where the Candida organism actually enters your bloodstream.

If not treated in time, this can become a deadly situation. You should understand that this usually only occurs when there is a severely compromised immune system present, such as cancer patients undergoing chemotherapy, or HIV/AIDS patients.

Q: Are There Over-The-Counter Medications They Clear up a Yeast Infection?

A: Candida overgrowth which presents itself as athlete's foot or a vaginal infection, or some other skin disorder, can be treated successfully with over-the-counter powers and creams.

If your Candida overgrowth becomes a chronic problem, it is going to create other symptoms and health concerns which require a more intensive treatment.

Q: What Natural or Holistic Remedies Are Available?

A: Essential oils can be used to effectively treat Candida. They may be dispersed into the air with an aromatherapy diffuser, or applied in a mixture directly to the skin. Lavender, magnesium, passion flower and chamomile are good for fighting Candida. Meditation has shown positive results in treating Candida.

So has exercise, which is a natural, holistic way to keep your immune system strong and your body healthy. Acupressure and acupuncture have shown promise as well. Ashwagandha and organic, potent, high quality black and green teas are effective for preventing and treating Candida.

Q: How Can I Change My Diet to Beat Candida?

A: A healthy body automatically keeps Candida in check. This means eating less fast foods, processed foods and sugar. Candida feeds on sugar. When you cut out fruit, milk, alcohol, peanuts, melons and other foods and beverages with sugar or yeast, your Candida will eventually starve. Eat leafier, green vegetables, choosing organic whenever you can.

You should avoid starchy vegetables like sweet potatoes and yams, peas, potatoes and carrots. Use nuts and berries as snack choices, instead of candy bars and sweets.

Coconut oil, Chia seeds and flaxseeds, turmeric and cinnamon spices, as well as sauerkraut and other fermented vegetables also provide a healthy platform for keeping Candida from getting out of control.

Final Thoughts

Candida is not just an irritating and painful inconvenience, it can also be life-threatening if its overgrowth and the damage it causes invade the blood stream and/or cause severe damage to the gastrointestinal tract. Fortunately, there are a lot of natural lifestyle measure you can take in what you wear, eat and drink that can help prevent Candida outbreaks from causing illness.

The best way to deal with Candida is to prevent it in the first place. If you have had one Candida infection, that is not unusual. But if you have frequent yeast infections, it is crucial to work with your doctor to discover the exact cause, so you can get the most effective treatment, and prevent any future outbreaks which can harm your health and ruin your quality of life.

To your best health!

Checklist: Foods to Avoid When Healing from Candida

When you are recovering from a Candida overgrowth and any resulting health issues, watching what you eat is vital to your recovery. This is because the best way to beat a fungal infection of Candida is to starve it. You simply don't give it the foods it needs to live, breed and multiply. Avoid eating the following foods when recovering from Candida overgrowth and your return to health will be quick and easy.

All types of sugar – Sugar is the preferred food of the Candida microorganism. Limit your consumption of sugar and you starve the overgrowth of Candida in your body. This includes artificial sweeteners, as well as the natural sugars found in honey and other foods.

Alcohol – Leaky gut syndrome is just one of multiple health problems related to alcohol consumption. Alcohol is hard on the linings of your intestines and can slow down your recovery.

Dairy products – A compromised gut is sensitive to the protein found in milk. This is the same for other dairy products, so they should be avoided while you are healing.

Fruit – You should normally be eating fruit regularly, but severely limit or entirely avoid it while healing your gut from Candida overgrowth. The natural fructose (sugar) found in fruits will slow down, or stop, your Candida recovery.

You may have limited quantities of low-fructose fruits like berries, limes, lemons and grapefruit, which possess healthy anti-microbial properties.

Starchy plant-based foods and vegetables – Steer clear of yams and sweet potatoes, other potatoes, beans, nuts, chickpeas and lentils.

Grains – Grains are forms of sugar, and should be avoided for this reason. If the grains contain gluten they can be extremely damaging to your gut health.

Coffee – Many coffee beans are high in mold and acidity. These can cause problems with your gut, which is extremely tender as you are healing from Candida overgrowth.

FODMAPS – Fermentable Oligo-, Di-, Monosaccharides and Polyols (FODMAPS) are carbohydrates which are not easily digested. These include cabbage, onions, apples and garlic, and should be avoided or at least limited while you are healing.

Bonus Tip: Foods to eat more of while healing:
- Coconut oil
- rutabaga
- seaweed
- ginger
- olive oil
- pumpkin seeds
- lemon and lime juice
- cayenne pepper

Other Relevant Books by This Author

If you would like to read more relevant books about this topic, here is a list of the CreateSpace links, titles and descriptions from this author:

https://www.createspace.com/6433160

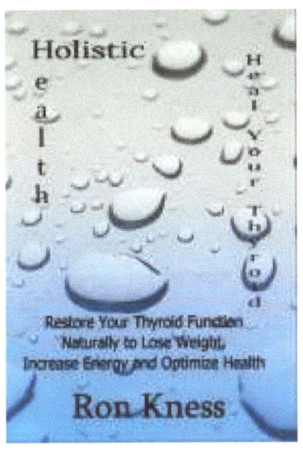

Heal Your Thyroid: Restore Your Thyroid Function Naturally to Lose Weight, Increase Energy and Optimize Health

The thyroid is a gland that is responsible for regulating many of your bodily functions and if it isn't functioning properly, you will experience a variety of symptoms that can impact your life in unfavorable ways.

The problem is that diagnosing a thyroid disorder can be difficult because the symptoms can be vague and attributed to many different things. Because of this, millions of people wake up every day with thyroid issues without even knowing it.

Do you constantly feel so fatigued that you barely have the energy to brush your teeth?

Do you find that there is more hair than usual ending up in your brush or shower drain?

Are you gaining weight or just not losing no matter how much you try to adapt a healthy lifestyle?

Do you often feel cold or have sensitivity to cold temperatures?

Do you have constant brain fog or memory issues?

Do you have dry eyes?

Well most of us experience these things at various times and because we simply assume that age is catching up with us or that we are not exercising as frequently as we should or that we are not getting enough sleep…we just chalk them up to something we have to live with and don't pursue any medical follow-up.

Many times it is an under-performing thyroid that is causing problems. With the proper nutrition, exercise and some lifestyle changes, you can heal your thyroid. They are all things you should be doing anyway, so what do you have to lose?

https://www.createspace.com/6528679

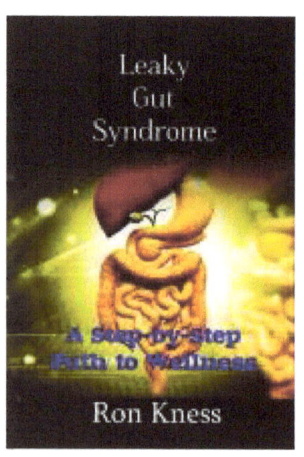

Leaky Gut Syndrome - Could This Be Why You Are Sick?: A Step-by-Step Path to Wellness

Leaky gut is just now starting to come onto the radar for doctors as more and more people are developing gastrointestinal and other disorders with no known cause. If you have frequent unexplained sickness, you could have leaky gut syndrome.

What it means is things are getting through the wall of the small intestine that aren't supposed to get through.

One of the big jobs of your small intestine is to finish the digestive process by continuing to break down the food you have eaten into smaller and smaller particles. And then, it absorbs the nutrients from that food through your intestinal wall and into your bloodstream where the nutrients can be absorbed by cells and converted into energy.

And it has another big job, too. It's supposed to keep harmful stuff inside the tube, where it can't cause too much trouble for your immune system. Things like bad germs, toxins, and food particles that are still too big for your body to use.

But sometimes, the lining of the small intestine gets damaged or the communication signals get confused resulting in things get through that shouldn't. And that can turn into even bigger problems in the form of infection or autoimmune disorders.

But in this guide, you will learn about what the leaky gut syndrome is, its potential causes, and proposed treatments that might be able to not only relieve your symptoms, but make leaky gut a thing of the past.

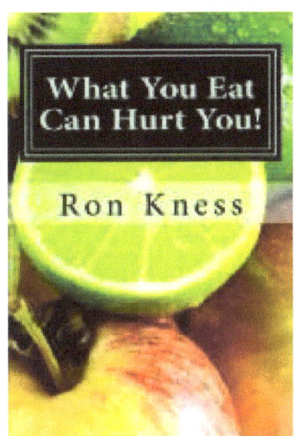

https://www.createspace.com/4963196

What You Eat Can Hurt You!: Learn Which Foods to Avoid and Which Ones to Eat to Stamp Out Inflammation, Illness and Disease, and to Stay Healthy!

Do you know that certain foods increase your risk for inflammation, disease and illness? It's true! And certain foods can help cure and heal you if you do get sick.

Knowing which foods to eat and which ones to avoid empowers you to manage your own health. After all, you have to look out for yourself.

Other topics discussed in this book are:
==> Health Mismanagement in Today's Society
==> Boost Your Health the Natural Way
==> Fight Disease with Proper Nutrition
==> Diabetic Nutritional Management
==> Prevent and Reverse Heart Disease the Natural Way
==> Take a Bite Out of Inflammation With Food
==> Remember, Nutrition Boosts Your Memory
==> News Flash - Control and Cure Cancer Through Nutrition
==> How to Cook Healthy

Take charge of your health today and learn which foods will keep you healthy and heal you, and which ones can make you sick or slow your healing. Click on the Buy Now with One Click button now and start reading in minutes how to maintain your health or get well.

About the Author

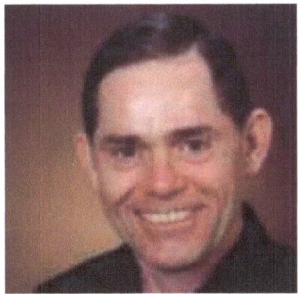

I have published over 125 books on Amazon for Kindle, CreateSpace and other publishing platforms.

While most of my books are on health and fitness in general, as I age (now 65) at the time of this writing) my topics of interest are geared toward aging baby boomers and older.

Besides my own writing, I also ghostwrite ebooks, books, reports, articles, blogs and do Kindle conversions for clients on a variety of topics.

Today my wife and I are retired from our careers and live in Gold Canyon, AZ. I now write as a retirement business where you'll find me happily sitting in my office typing away on my laptop as I work on my next book or ghostwriting project . . . that is if we are not traveling on a cruise ship - our new-found mode of travel.

www.ingramcontent.com/pod-product-compliance
Lightning Source LLC
Chambersburg PA
CBHW050829290526
45792CB00001B/324